Prescription for Success

A Roadmap to Limitless Opportunities

Shadawn Henderson

ISBN: 979-8-9876247-6-0

IF I CAN, SO CAN YOU!

Prescription for Success

A Roadmap to Limitless Opportunities

Shadawn Henderson

Dedication Page

This book is first and foremost devoted to my Lord and Savior, Jesus Christ. It is because of you that I not only enjoy writing, but also want to inspire others. My Lord, I appreciate you for this adventure and eagerly await where you will take me next. I also dedicate this book to my parents, who have always been supportive of my endeavors. I adore you!

Table of Contents

Note

Welcome to the electrifying world of pharmacy, where dreams come alive, and futures are forged! Prepare to embark on a thrilling journey that will not only shape your career, but also define the very essence of who you are as a person.

Congratulations are in order, for you have boldly chosen the path less traveled, fueled by an unwavering passion for pharmaceutical excellence. Your commitment and determination have led you here, and now it's time to seize the opportunity to make an impact in the world. Reflect, dear reader, on the profound reasons that guided you to this momentous decision. Contemplate the lives you will touch, the communities you will empower, and the legacy you will leave behind.

Yes, this is your time to shine! Amidst the trials and tribulations of this arduous journey, you may have relinquished certain desires that others freely indulge in.

Yet, know this: nothing worth having comes without sacrifice. Rest assured, every ounce of dedication poured into your pursuits will blossom into a radiant testament of success, surpassing the mere acquisition of material possessions. So, brace yourself, for within these pages lies a treasure trove of wisdom, insights, and invaluable knowledge, waiting to be gleaned. It's time to unlock the secrets that will propel you to new heights in the realm of pharmacy.

Embrace this exhilarating adventure and wield the power to heal, to transform lives, and to shape the future of healthcare. The rewards that await you are beyond measure. **Believe in yourself**, trust in your abilities, and remember, the journey you're about to embark upon is a sacred calling destined to fulfill your wildest aspirations.

Get ready to blossom into the exceptional pharmacist you were always meant to become. Your future awaits – it's time to take the leap!

Good Luck DOCTOR!!!

Introduction

Whether you are a first-generation student interested in pursuing a career in pharmacy or an experienced professional seeking a new outlook, this book serves as your gateway to a prosperous future in the field. Within its contents, you will uncover a plethora of information regarding the diverse aspects of pharmacy, providing you with a strong groundwork for your professional journey.

From prerequisite courses and undergraduate requirements to gaining valuable patient experience, we'll guide you every step of the way. But the road to pharmacy school doesn't end there. Learn how to stand out from the crowd with brilliant personal statements that captivate admissions committees. Craft compelling letters of recommendation and present your transcripts with confidence.

Explore the realm of supplemental essays and discover the key to securing your desired position in the program of your dreams. Get ready to impress during admission interviews by refining your abilities through practice and discovering the fundamental principles that resonate with your vision of achievement. As you delve into different pharmacy schools, you will unearth crucial information that will drive you to dive deeper into researching your potential institutions. This will allow you to gain a better understanding of how each school provides a distinctive learning atmosphere, empowering you to customize your education according to your needs.

With a treasure trove of potential interview questions at your fingertips, you'll outshine the competition and articulate your passion for the field. Discover insider tips and strategies that will leave a lasting impression on interviewers and showcase your intellectual and physical preparedness like never before. Once you've secured your place, look into the world of scholarships, financial aid, and living arrangements near your chosen school. Gain insights into the indispensable role of social media etiquette and explore the myriad career pathways available to pharmacy graduates.

The possibilities are endless, and this book will open your eyes to a future brimming with opportunities. Say yes to a rewarding career in pharmacy.

Uncover the secrets, seize the opportunities, and unlock your true potential. Your journey starts here.

I. You Are Fearfully and Wonderfully Made

1.   What Is Pharmacy?

So, you've decided to pursue a career in pharmacy! How did you get here? Do you come from a line of medical professionals? Are your parents, themselves pharmacists?

Maybe, you are first generation, like me! Congratulations to you all for deciding to pursue such a rewarding journey with endless opportunities, especially if you are first generation.

Pharmacy is a multifaceted profession that blends science, health care, technology, ethics, and business. It's like you get the best of both worlds here. Pharmacy entails the cultivation of drug-producing plants, the synthesis of chemical compounds, and the examination of medicinal agents.

Since 1683, the pharmaceutical business has evolved, and with your drive, this industry will continue to do so! When people consider pursuing a career in pharmacy, the first thing that usually comes to mind are their local community pharmacists dispensing medications and providing healthcare advice. While community pharmacy is a rewarding career pathway, it is not the only option for pharmacists!

Discover the hidden world of pharmacy career pathways as you embark on an eye-opening journey of knowledge. Unveil diverse and intriguing pharmacy practice and specialty roles that will astonish even the most seasoned pharmacy enthusiasts. Unravel the tapestry of endless opportunities that lie within the realm of pharmacy careers and allow yourself the opportunity to explore the boundless possibilities that await you. Prepare to be captivated by the abundance of choices and propel your dreams to new heights in the captivating world of pharmacy.

2. Pharmacy School Requirements

You never know what a school is looking for in an applicant! You may be a stellar student, the captain of the baseball, chess, or other teams, an active community volunteer, have shadowing hours, and have absolutely everything a school looks for in a prospective applicant and still not get accepted! Then there's me. One who has retaken classes (MY GOODNESS), is still connected in my impoverished neighborhood through shadowing hours, and so on, but has a KILLER personal statement attached to a meaningful story! As I began my application process, I had no idea how many schools to apply to, what institutions look for in potential applicants, or whether I really had a chance at pharmacy school, but that's where my faith came in.

I'd been debating whether I was cut out for pharmacy school when I chose to attend UC Davis' Pre-Health Conference (highly recommended). I knew by attending, I'd be able to introduce myself to some of the admissions team members while also sharing my "why". It was critical for me to discuss my circumstances and the gravity of my decision to study pharmacy. I may have had a challenging start to higher education, having several W's on my college transcript, and having to retake classes, but I knew I was more than just grades. Not only did I have an increasing trend, but I also possessed a master's degree.

I'd also published research on direct oral anticoagulants and vitamin-K antagonist and had many years of experience in other fields. Going to this conference, I knew I had to be prepared, and I was! I recommend that you not only attend but also customize your CV (more on that later). Bring something that will allow you to stand out! I printed out my CV, publication, and brought business cards, since it was critical to me that the committee put a face to my name.

This was my third time attending, but the first as a potential pharmacy student! With hundreds of booths, recruiters, and students, I knew I'd leave with the answer I was looking for! **Was pharmacy school right for me?** I utilized this chance to be honest, truthful, and open to constructive criticism. My story was important, therefore I made sure admission committees knew it as well!

With a bachelor's and master's degree in biomedical sciences, I knew I had almost all the necessary prerequisites, especially since the PCAT (Pharmacy College Admission Test) was no longer required! Depending on the pharmacy school, some common course prerequisites could include:

- Biostatistics may be desired or necessary.
- Social/Behavioral Science: Psychology and/or sociology may be necessary.
- Humanities courses, including history, philosophy, literature, and religion, may be required.
- English Composition: Required.
- Public speaking and communication skills may be desirable or necessary.
- Microbiology.
- Biology/Biological Sciences: Most courses need General Biology I and II. Cell biology and genetics may also be accepted or necessary.
- Some schools accept distinct anatomy and physiology courses, while others mix A&P I and II.
- Commonly required chemistry courses include general and organic chemistry I and II.
- Physics
- Calculus: Highly recommended.

Lab requirements for the above courses may vary.

Despite having the necessary credentials, my path into healthcare was not straightforward, which made me hesitant. I believe it is critical for you, as a reader, to know and grasp this! I did not have a 4.0, I grew up in an underserved single-parent household, worked my way through college, and spent 5 years at a community college before transferring to a 4-year university, simply because having an income and a social life were my primary goals. I should mention that I had shifted from being a pre-med student (more on that later).

Note, most schools demand successful completion of academic coursework before admission. In fact, required course requirements can be in process when you submit your application and planned after you submit it. However, all prerequisites must be successfully finished in the year in which one plans to enter the program.

Keep in mind the required prerequisite courses do not represent the total number of semester hours pharmacy applicants must finish for each topic. For more information on specific programs, please visit the PharmCas School Directory.

3.   No One-Size-Fits-All to Obtaining a PharmD

There is no one-size-fits-all approach to obtaining a PharmD degree, as the path can vary depending on your background and your academic standing. Different colleges and pharmacy schools may have their own unique program structures and lengths, which can work to your advantage. Once you have successfully completed all the required pre-pharmacy coursework, you will enter the professional phase of the PharmD curriculum. The specific pre-pharmacy coursework may differ from institution to institution, but it is possible to enter a program with various structures. These structures may include early assurance, 2–3-year, 3–4-year, 4 years, and 6–7-year programs.

PharmD programs and early assurance programs are coupled, enabling students to enroll within a year or two of starting college. They move swiftly into the professional phase after fulfilling the pre-pharmacy requirements. Traditional applicants are encouraged by pharmacy schools.

Accelerated 2-3-year programs are usually intended for individuals who hold a bachelor's degree in a related profession. Students can earn a PharmD degree faster thanks to these programs, which compress the necessary courses into a shorter period. Students who have fulfilled some of the prerequisites already or who wish to enter the workforce sooner may find this useful.

The most popular route to a PharmD degree is a 3-4-year program. Students who have finished the required pre-pharmacy coursework and are prepared to move on to the professional part of the curriculum are the target audience for these programs. Three years are usually allotted to the coursework, with advanced pharmacy practice experiences (APPEs) in a variety of healthcare settings making up the last year.

Like 3-4-year programs, 4-year programs could have extra requirements or courses. These courses could be more rigorous or provide more chances for research or specialization. Students who wish to focus on areas of pharmacy or who are considering further education or research options in the future may find them to be a good fit.

Students who want to complete both their undergraduate and PharmD degrees in a combined program can apply to 6- or 7-year programs. These programs usually enable students to fulfill the prerequisite pre-pharmacy coursework in addition to earning their bachelor's degree in a relevant discipline. Students can easily move from their undergraduate studies into the professional portion of the PharmD program.

The duration and structure of a PharmD program can vary depending on the school and the student's academic achievements. It is important to explore different program options to find the best fit for your goals.

4. *Notes*

Prescription for Success

Notes

Prescription for Success

Notes

Prescription for Success

Notes

Prescription for Success

Notes

Prescription for Success

II. He Will Never Leave nor Forsake You

5.   Curriculum Vitae

You may be familiar with the resume—a brief document used largely for industrial job applications—during your professional career. However, it is critical to consider the comprehensive documenting of your academic achievements and experiences. A curriculum vitae (CV) is a thorough dossier that meticulously documents your whole academic history. A CV, as opposed to a resume, is a comprehensive record that should include a detailed description of your educational background, work history, scholarly publications, and formal presentations, as well as any applicable certifications and internships completed.

In addition, a CV should include any voluntary initiatives completed and provide a summary of the awards and honors throughout your educational and professional endeavors. The primary goal of a CV is to promote and celebrate your academic achievements; so, it requires a focus on those accomplishments to enhance your profile in a competitive field of candidates.

Furthermore, the ongoing curation and refining of your CV serves a variety of functions. It makes it easier to write a captivating personal statement—a story that clearly and persuasively expresses your motives and qualifications. In the world of work, a well-maintained and comprehensive CV can be the key to unlocking opportunities, giving you a major edge when applying for jobs or internships. Also, for those entering the pharmaceutical industry, such a document becomes an essential tool for navigating the Pharmacy College Application Service (PharmCAS) portal.

As a result, you must devote time and effort to creating and updating your CV on a continuous basis. The discipline necessary to maintain this document reflects your commitment to your academic and professional lives, ultimately moving you toward your intended career goals. The length of one's CV varies according to their experiences. Understanding how to format a CV will allow you to develop a captivating and impressionable document.

Here are some basic steps for writing a CV:

1. Header

   Include your name, phone number, and email address at the top of your CV for easy identification and contact.

2. Education

   In reverse chronological order, list your educational history, highlighting degrees obtained and those in progress.

3. Work Experience

   Provide a comprehensive account of your employment history, such as full-time/part-time roles, internships, and research activities. For each role, specify your job title, employer, location, employment period, and a brief description of responsibilities.

4. Additional Sections

   Expand your CV with any relevant achievements, which may consist of publications, presentations, community involvement, grants, awards, professional memberships, and conference participation, certifications, among others.

5. Personal Interests

   Optionally, you may mention hobbies or interests that might resonate with the role or organization.

Here's a basic template you can use when making your CV:

[Your Name]
[Contact]
[Email Address]

Education
[Title of Degree] [Dates Attended]
[School Name]

Employment
[*Job Title*] [Dates of Employment]
[Name of Employer] [City and State of the Employer]
[Describe your Responsibilities]

Research Experience
[Type of Research] [Date]
[Description of your Duties].

Publications
[Authors Highlighting your Name in Bold] [Year of Publication] [Title of Article] [Publishing Journal]

Volunteer Experience
[*Position or Job Performed*] [Date of Service]
[Organization] [City and State of the Organization]
[Accomplishment]

Academic Achievements
[Name of Award] [Year]

Certifications
[Name of Certification] [Year]

6.   Applying to Pharmacy School

The initial step in the process of applying to pharmacy school involves creating an account on PharmCas. After successfully doing so, you will receive your CAS ID number, which should be kept in a readily accessible location in case it is needed. If you find yourself in a situation where you require assistance with transcripts or navigating the website, you may need to contact PharmCas, as I have done. For individuals from underserved communities who are first-generation students, or those who are unfamiliar with PharmCas, the initial navigation may be challenging, but with time, you will become more comfortable.

Now that you have set up your account, let us proceed to the next step, which involves reviewing your application dashboard. This dashboard will grant you access to all the necessary sections of the application, allowing you to have a comprehensive overview of your progress. As you work through each section of the application, it is important to take notes, gather all the required documents, and remember that until you receive an acceptance, PharmCas is your best friend.

1. *Personal Information*

This section is uncomplicated and direct. The details you provide here are utilized to collect your biographical and contact information, along with your citizenship, race/ethnicity, and other family details. It is important to be honest!

2. *Academic History*

It is necessary to include a list of all schools you have attended, starting with high school. After that, you should list any colleges you have attended, provide transcript entries, and include scores from standardized tests if applicable. It is important to order official transcripts for yourself and to have them sent to PharmCas. Transcripts can be sent either electronically or by mail. Please note that PharmCas only accepts transcripts from Parchment and the National Student Clearinghouse.

If you are currently in high school and plan to apply to pharmacy school in the future, it is recommended that you start a folder or file to keep all your important academic papers. It is also important to note that the PCAT (Pharmacy College Admissions Test) is no longer a requirement for admission acceptance. In fact, many institutions have removed the PCAT from their admission criteria. If you still intend to take the PCAT, I suggest registering for the exam several months before the submission deadline for your test scores.

Submitting accurate information to your chosen schools is one of the most crucial steps in the application process. Your academic transcripts play a key role in providing precise information. They serve as official documentation of your enrollment, courses, and grades from any previous educational institution where you have obtained credits or taken exams.

These documents may originate from medical schools, vocational schools, or universities. It is crucial to possess accurate and up-to-date transcripts as selection committees evaluate them alongside your personal statement and letters of recommendation to determine your preparedness for the study and practice. While each institution may have slightly different requirements, typically, an official transcript is stamped with the school's seal and the registrar's signature and is delivered in a sealed envelope. However, some schools may electronically send official transcripts through a system like eSCRIP-SAFE.

This process involves creating a secure digital file that is then transmitted to a program for expedited delivery to the recipient. It is essential to never tamper with a sealed transcript envelope under any circumstances. Whether utilizing a physical or digital record, it is important to meticulously track and document when your transcripts have been sent to and received by PharmCas and your designated programs. Nowadays, many students can easily monitor a significant portion of the verification process through their application portals, allowing them to confirm successful delivery.

Upon receipt, you will receive a notification of receipt from PharmCas. PharmCas offers a paid service to have someone input your grades, or you can do it yourself. It is important to note that your file will not be verified or released to your prospective institution until PharmCas has received all transcripts. You will be unable to input grades from your transcript if your attended colleges section is incomplete.

To ensure accurate completion of the transcript entry section, it is important to report all courses listed on your transcripts. This includes courses from which you withdrew, repeated courses, ungraded courses, and so forth. When listing your courses, make sure to categorize them under the correct term, year, and class level. Department prefixes and course numbers should match exactly as they appear on your transcripts.

Courses should be entered under the institution where they were originally taken, following the format on the original school's transcript. This applies even if the courses were transferred to another institution or taken during high school for college credit. Include all in-progress and planned courses, along with all completed courses up to the current date. Upon completion of these steps, you will have the opportunity to review and finalize your transcripts.

3. *Supporting Information*

This section is used to collect supporting application information, such as evaluations (letters of recommendations), experiences, achievements, licenses, and certifications, and finally, your personal statement.

Evaluations

All evaluations, in the form of letters of recommendation (LOR's), must be submitted electronically by the evaluators themselves through PharmCas's recommender portal, Liaison Letters, unless the school you are applying to specifies otherwise. I would advise you to be cautious when selecting individuals to write your LOR. The LOR's you receive, whether from an academic professor, medical professional, or employer, can have a significant impact on your application. For example, if you are performing poorly in a professor's class, it would not be wise to approach them for an evaluation. Similarly, if you consistently arrive late to work, it is highly unlikely that you would ask your employer for an evaluation. If you believe that your potential evaluator does not have anything positive to say about you or your work ethic, it is best not to ask them. The application process is already extensive and expensive, so we want to avoid applying multiple cycles. It is important to inform your evaluators about the application process and provide them with a deadline. Once you request evaluations, your evaluator will receive an email with a link to Liaison Letters, where they can review your request and either accept, complete, or decline it. You will be notified once your evaluation is finished. Committee letters are also accepted. You have the option to request up to 4 evaluations, so choose wisely.

Experiences

Let us discuss experiences. Within this section, you can input your professional experiences across various categories or types. It is crucial that you exercise your best judgment when categorizing your experiences to determine the appropriate category. If you are uncertain, it is advisable to seek guidance from your prospective program or contact PharmCas. PharmCas recommends focusing on experiences within the past 10 years, particularly those at or above the collegiate level. Examples of experience types include pharmacy experience, healthcare experience, any form of employment, as well as extracurricular or volunteer experience. It is of utmost importance that you provide information about the organization and supervisor, as this greatly influences the verification process. Your CV should assist you in pulling the relevant date range for each experience to be entered in this section. Additionally, ensure that you provide concise details about each experience in your own words. Tools such as Grammarly can aid in refining your job duties description for brevity.

Here is one example from of my experiences:

In terms of my experience in the healthcare sector, I have mentioned T'ena Health, a non-profit organization that I actively participated in. The primary objective of this organization is to eliminate health disparities. As for the details of my role and responsibilities there, it includes:

"My duties with T'ena consists of planning and attending free community health fairs as well as distributing hygiene kits. T'ena highlighted the shortage of health care workers in marginalized places, as well as the consequences of rural health inequities. T'ena gave me the opportunity to canvas and engage with the unsheltered to create relationships with people who are homeless. I discovered a compassionate method to resolving health inequities by providing resources tailored to the individual."

In my academic journey, I encountered some challenges that were crucial for me to address. It was essential for me to highlight experiences that not only sparked my passion but also resonated with the mission of the school I was applying to. Understanding the mission of each school is imperative. It is advisable to engage in experiences that you can speak about with enthusiasm, especially during interviews. Merely listing an experience to fulfill a requirement is not recommended. It is highly recommended to complete this section on PharmCas for various reasons, primarily to showcase your unique experiences. Market yourself effectively! Please note that once you submit your application, you will not be able to edit previously entered experiences if you have provided both start and end dates. However, you can add new experiences and update ongoing ones. Additionally, you will need to specify the average number of hours per week dedicated to each experience within the indicated date range, so honesty is key.

The highest number of hours I recorded for a single experience was 11,936 hours. While this may seem like a significant amount, it was due to my full-time role in retail where I worked 32 hours per week for a total of 373 weeks. Despite this position not being directly related to the medical field, it was my initial exposure to customer service, from which I gained valuable skills applicable to pharmacy school. I honed my customer service abilities, set weekly sales targets, analyzed sales data, collaborated with merchandising, provided training to staff, and delivered efficient customer service. This experience taught me discipline, resilience, and how to handle rejection. Moreover, it emphasized the importance of understanding customer needs, building connections, and overcoming communication barriers.

Achievements

Ever since embarking on my health journey, I have achieved several milestone accomplishments. Firstly, I was fortunate to obtain a scholarship that has supported me throughout my academic pursuits. Additionally, I have successfully published a scientific article (thanks Dr. Tran), showcasing my contributions to the field of science. Furthermore, I have established a book publishing company which has allowed me to indulge in my passion for self-publishing. These achievements not only highlight my dedication and commitment but also demonstrate my ability to pursue diverse interests beyond academia.

Therefore, I encourage you to share your own accomplishments along your journey, as it is an excellent platform to showcase your personal interests and talents. The committee welcomes all relevant professional or academic achievements, which can be categorized into various types such as honors, scholarships, or publications. Choose the category that best aligns with your accomplishments and accolades.

Licenses and Certifications

Adding professional licenses or certifications that you have acquired is always a wise choice. While this section will not be verified, it still holds significance. It is important to note that you can only list current licenses and certifications, as the system does not permit the entry of past valid credentials.

Personal Statements

Why Pharmacy?

How does the acquisition of a Doctor of Pharmacy degree align with your immediate and long-term career aspirations?

The initial two inquiries should serve as a starting point for you to contemplate the concept of constructing your personal statement. Your personal statement should reflect your own motivations and reasons. As I began crafting my personal statement, I conducted a thorough self-assessment. I compiled a list of at least 16 topics on a piece of paper that I could expand upon. These topics ranged from experiences in my childhood, including instances of trauma, to the development of my passion for the profession. This is how I formulated my personal statement. In your personal statement, it is advisable to initially approach the essay topic in a broad manner. Although there is a character limit, as you revise your essay, you will gradually condense your writing. You have likely heard the phrase "show but don't tell" when discussing personal statements, and it holds truth. Similarly, the opening paragraph of your personal statement should captivate the reader's attention. By following these two steps alone, not only will you pique the committee's interest in reading your entire essay, but you will also leave them wanting to learn more about you.

Remember, your story is significant, so utilize this opportunity to truly shine. Make sure to thoroughly proofread your essay multiple times to identify any grammatical or punctuation errors before submitting it. Additionally, if possible, seek feedback from a few trustworthy individuals who can review your personal statement. Once you submit your application, you will be unable to make any further edits, so please keep this in mind. Overall, I outlined how my personal, educational, and professional experiences will enhance my ability to be a culturally sensitive and competent pharmacist, ultimately leading to an improvement in the quality of life for all individuals, particularly those in marginalized communities.

4. *Program Materials*

Lastly, it is crucial to think about the school you have chosen. While selecting a school to apply to may seem straightforward, it is important to understand the reasons behind your choice. You should ensure that the institution you are considering is a place where you can envision yourself for the next 3-4 years. Several factors should be considered, including the mission statement of the institution. **Do your personal values align with theirs?** What are the significant questions to ask if you are granted an interview? With so many pharmacy schools available, it is essential to narrow down your options.

In my case, my parents have been my greatest support, and I knew that obtaining a doctorate degree would not be an easy journey. Therefore, staying close to home was a priority for me. As I began researching potential schools, there were a few key factors that held great significance for me. One of them was the percentage of underserved acceptances each year. Being an African American woman and a first-generation student from an underserved background, this was particularly important to me.

Additionally, the class sizes and student-to-teacher ratio were crucial considerations for me, as education can be quite expensive. I needed to know what resources would be available to support my success (this responsibility also falls on you).

Moreover, the first-time NAPLEX pass rates and Residency Match Rates held significant importance to me.

By conducting thorough research on your prospective program, you can further narrow down your choices. Furthermore, it is worth mentioning that applications can be costly, so do not hesitate to reach out to the institution and inquire about potential fee waivers.

7.   Pharmacy Schools by State

Below you will see a list of colleges categorized by state, providing you with a wide range of options to choose from. Each state offers its own unique advantages and opportunities, so it is important to carefully consider the location of the schools you are interested in.

One factor to consider is the climate of the state. If you prefer warmer weather, states like California, Florida, or Texas may be more appealing to you. On the other hand, if you enjoy the changing seasons and colder temperatures, states like New York, Massachusetts, or Colorado might be a better fit.

Another consideration is the cost of living in each state. Some states, such as New York or California, have a higher cost of living compared to others. This can impact your overall expenses while attending school, including housing, groceries, and transportation. It is important to factor in these costs when making your decision.

Additionally, the location of the school can also impact your access to internships, job opportunities, and networking events. Certain states, like California or New York, are known for their thriving industries and job markets. If you are interested in pursuing a specific career path, it may be beneficial to choose a school located in a state that offers ample opportunities in that field.

Furthermore, the cultural and social aspects of each state should also be considered. Different states have their own unique traditions, customs, and lifestyles. If you are looking for a specific cultural experience or want to immerse yourself in a particular community, it is important to research the state and city where the school is located.

Ultimately, the location of the institution should align with your personal preferences, goals, and aspirations. It is important to take the time to research and visit the schools you are considering getting a better sense of the environment and determine if it is the right fit for you.

By considering the schools' locations as a major factor in your decision-making process, you can ensure that you choose a school that not only offers a quality education but also provides an environment that supports your personal and academic growth.

- **Alabama**
    - Auburn University Harrison College of Pharmacy
    - Samford University McWhorter School of Pharmacy

- **Arizona**
    - Midwestern University – Glendale College of Pharmacy
    - University of Arizona R. Ken Coit College of Pharmacy

- **Arkansas**
    - Harding University College of Pharmacy
    - University of Arkansas for Medical Sciences College of Pharmacy

- **California**
    - American University of Health Sciences School of Pharmacy
    - California Health Sciences University College of Pharmacy
    - California Northstate University College of Pharmacy
    - Chapman University School of Pharmacy
    - Keck Graduate Institute School of Pharmacy and Health Sciences
    - Loma Linda University School of Pharmacy
    - Marshall B. Ketchum University College of Pharmacy
    - Touro University – California College of Pharmacy
    - University of California, Irvine School of Pharmacy
    - University of California, San Diego Skaggs School of Pharmacy
    - University of California, San Francisco School of Pharmacy
    - University of Southern California Alfred E. Mann School of Pharmacy

- University of the Pacific Thomas J. Long School of Pharmacy
- West Coast University School of Pharmacy
- Western University of Health Sciences College of Pharmacy

- **Colorado**
  - Regis University Rueckert – Hartman College for Health Professions School of Pharmacy
  - University of Colorado Anschutz Medical Campus Skaggs School of Pharmacy

- **Connecticut**
  - University of Connecticut School of Pharmacy
  - University of Saint Joseph School of Pharmacy

- **District of Columbia**
  - Howard University College of Pharmacy

- **Florida**
  - Florida A&M University College of Pharmacy
  - Larkin University College of Pharmacy
  - Nova Southeastern University Barry and Judy Silverman College of Pharmacy
  - Palm Beach Atlantic University Lloyd L. Gregory School of Pharmacy
  - University of Florida College of Pharmacy
  - University of South Florida Health Taneja College of Pharmacy

- **Georgia**
  - Mercer University College of Pharmacy
  - Philadelphia College of Osteopathic Medicine – Georgia School of Pharmacy
  - South University School of Pharmacy
  - University of Georgia College of Pharmacy

- **Hawaii**

- University of Hawaii at Hilo Daniel K. Inouye College of Pharmacy

- **Idaho**
  - Idaho State University L.S. Skaggs College of Pharmacy

- **Illinois**
  - Chicago State University College of Health Sciences and Pharmacy
  - Midwestern University College of Pharmacy
  - Roosevelt University College of Science, Health, and Pharmacy
  - Rosalind Franklin University of Medicine and Science College of Pharmacy
  - Southern Illinois University Edwardsville School of Pharmacy
  - University of Illinois at Chicago College of Pharmacy

- **Indiana**
  - Butler University College of Pharmacy and Health Sciences
  - Manchester University College of Pharmacy, Natural and Health Sciences
  - Purdue University College of Pharmacy

- **International**
  - Lebanese American University School of Pharmacy

- **Iowa**
  - Drake University College of Pharmacy and Health Sciences
  - University of Iowa College of Pharmacy

- **Kansas**
  - University of Kansas School of Pharmacy

- **Kentucky**

- Sullivan University College of Pharmacy and Health Sciences
- University of Kentucky College of Pharmacy

- **Louisiana**
  - University of Louisiana and Monroe College of Pharmacy
  - Xavier University of Louisiana College of Pharmacy

- **Maine**
  - Husson University College of Health and Pharmacy School of Pharmacy
  - University of New England Westbrook College of Health Professions School of Pharmacy

- **Maryland**
  - Notre Dame of Maryland University School of Pharmacy
  - University of Maryland School of Pharmacy
  - University of Maryland Eastern Shore School of Pharmacy and Health Professions

- **Massachusetts**
  - Massachusetts College of Pharmacy and Health Sciences – Worcester
  - Massachusetts College of Pharmacy and Health Sciences – Boston
  - Northeastern University Bouvé College of Health Sciences School of Pharmacy and Pharmaceutical Sciences
  - Western New England University College of Pharmacy and Health Sciences

- **Michigan**
  - Ferris State University College of Pharmacy
  - University of Michigan College of Pharmacy
  - Wayne State University Eugene Applebaum College of Pharmacy and Health Sciences

- **Minnesota**
  - University of Minnesota College of Pharmacy

- **Mississippi**
  - University of Mississippi School of Pharmacy
  - William Carey University School of Pharmacy

- **Missouri**
  - University of Health Sciences and Pharmacy in St. Louis – St. Louis College of Pharmacy
  - University of Missouri – Kansas City School of Pharmacy

- **Montana**
  - University of Montana College of Health Skaggs School of Pharmacy

- **Nebraska**
  - Creighton University School of Pharmacy and Health Professions
  - University of Nebraska Medical Center College of Pharmacy

- **Nevada**
  - Roseman University of Health Sciences College of Pharmacy

- **New Jersey**
  - Fairleigh Dickinson University School of Pharmacy and Health Sciences
  - Rutgers Ernest Mario School of Pharmacy

- **New Mexico**
  - University of New Mexico College of Pharmacy

- **New York**
  - Albany College of Pharmacy and Health Sciences
  - Binghamton University State of New York School of Pharmacy and Pharmaceutical Sciences

- D'Youville University School of Pharmacy
- Long Island University Arnold and Marie Schwartz College of Pharmacy and Health Sciences
- St. John Fisher University Wegmans School of Pharmacy
- St. John's University College of Pharmacy and Health Sciences
- Touro College of Pharmacy – NY
- University at Buffalo Pharmacy and Pharmaceutical Sciences

- **North Carolina**
  - Campbell University College of Pharmacy and Health Sciences
  - High Point University Fred Wilson School of Pharmacy
  - Wingate University School of Pharmacy

- **North Dakota**
  - North Dakota State University School of Pharmacy

- **Ohio**
  - Cedarville University School of Pharmacy
  - Northeast Ohio Medical University College of Pharmacy
  - Ohio Northern University Raabe College of Pharmacy
  - Ohio State University College of Pharmacy
  - University of Cincinnati James L. Winkle College of Pharmacy
  - University of Findlay College of Pharmacy
  - University of Toledo College of Pharmacy and Pharmaceutical Sciences

- **Oklahoma**
  - Southwestern Oklahoma State University College of Pharmacy
  - University of Oklahoma Health Sciences Center College of Pharmacy

- **Oregon**
  - Oregon State University College of Pharmacy

- Pacific University School of Pharmacy

- **Pennsylvania**
  - Duquesne University School of Pharmacy
  - Lake Erie College of Osteopathic Medicine School of Pharmacy
  - Saint Joseph's University Philadelphia College of Pharmacy
  - Temple University School of Pharmacy
  - Thomas Jefferson University Jefferson College of Pharmacy
  - University of Pittsburgh School of Pharmacy
  - Wilkes University Nesbitt School of Pharmacy

- **Puerto Rico**
  - University of Puerto Rico Medical Science Campus School of Pharmacy

- **Rhode Island**
  - University of Rhode Island College of Pharmacy

- **South Carolina**
  - Medical University of South Carolina College of Pharmacy
  - Presbyterian College School of Pharmacy
  - South Carolina College of Pharmacy
  - University of South Carolina College of Pharmacy

- **South Dakota**
  - South Dakota State University College of Pharmacy and Allied Health Professions

- **Tennessee**
  - Belmont University College of Pharmacy and Health Sciences
  - East Tennessee State University Bill Gatton College of Pharmacy

- Lipscomb University Health Sciences Center College of Pharmacy
- South College School of Pharmacy
- Union University College of Pharmacy
- University of Tennessee Health Science Center College of Pharmacy

- **Texas**
  - Texas A&M University Health Sciences Center Irma Lerma Rangel School of Pharmacy
  - Texas Southern University Joan M. Lafleur College of Pharmacy and Health Sciences
  - Texas Tech University Health Sciences Center Jerry H. Hodge School of Pharmacy
  - University of Houston College of Pharmacy
  - University of North Texas Health Sciences UNT System College of Pharmacy
  - University of Texas at Austin College of Pharmacy
  - University of Texas at El Paso School of Pharmacy
  - University of Texas at Tyler Ben and Maytee Fisch College of Pharmacy
  - University of the Incarnate Word Feik School of Pharmacy

- **Utah**
  - University of Utah College of Pharmacy

- **Virginia**
  - Appalachian College of Pharmacy
  - Hampton University School of Pharmacy
  - Shenandoah University Bernard J. Dunn School of Pharmacy
  - Virginia Commonwealth University at the Medical College of Virginia Campus School of Pharmacy

- **Washington**
  - University of Washington School of Pharmacy

- Washington State University College of Pharmacy and Pharmaceutical Sciences

- **West Virginia**
  - Marshall University School of Pharmacy
  - University of Charleston School of Pharmacy
  - West Virginia University School of Pharmacy

- **Wisconsin**
  - Concordia University Wisconsin School of Pharmacy
  - Medical College of Wisconsin School of Pharmacy
  - University of Wisconsin-Madison School of Pharmacy

- **Wyoming**
  - University of Wyoming School of Pharmacy

8. Notes

Prescription for Success

Notes

Prescription for Success

Notes

Prescription for Success

Notes

Prescription for Success

Notes

Prescription for Success

III.   Have Faith the Size of a Mustard Seed

9.   Social Media Etiquette

Maintaining a positive and professional online presence can also enhance one's chances of securing internships, job opportunities, and networking with potential mentors in the pharmacy industry. By consistently showcasing a commitment to professionalism and ethical behavior on social media platforms, aspiring pharmacy students can build a strong reputation and credibility within the field.

In addition, utilizing social media platforms to stay updated on current trends, research, and advancements in the pharmacy industry can also be beneficial for aspiring pharmacy students. By following reputable pharmacy organizations, journals, and professionals on social media, students can gain valuable insights and knowledge that can help them excel in their academic and professional pursuits.

Overall, while social media can be a valuable tool for aspiring pharmacy students to connect with others in the field and showcase their passion for pharmacy, it is crucial to always prioritize professionalism, respect, and ethical behavior in all online interactions. By doing so, students can effectively leverage social media to enhance their academic and professional growth in the pharmacy industry.

10. Preparing for Admission Interviews

1. *Do Your Research!*

The question of "Why did you choose us?" is undoubtedly one that you will encounter, and it necessitates a sincere and genuine response. It is crucial to be well-prepared for a pharmacy school interview by understanding the reasons behind your choice of the school you are applying to. Thorough research on your prospective school is essential. This research should encompass various aspects such as academics, accreditation, tuition fees, and even the curriculum if you are inclined to do so. Additionally, it is important to gather information about the school's academic calendar system (semester, quarter, or block) and the duration of the program. It is also beneficial to explore the attrition rate and any other factors related to student achievements.

During my own exploration of pharmacy schools, I reached out to current students through social media platforms to gain insights into the school's atmosphere. Hearing feedback from both current and past students is an excellent way to understand the overall experience. The American Association of Colleges of Pharmacy (AACP) offers a valuable online directory called the "Pharmacy School Admissions Requirements," which provides comprehensive information about all AACP recognized pharmacy schools in the United States and Canada. This resource, which is accessible for free, includes detailed profiles, statistics, and other valuable information that can assist you in comprehending what each school has to offer. The profiles cover a wide range of topics, including admission requirements, selection factors, and tuition fees.

Furthermore, it is advisable to familiarize yourself with the faculty members of your prospective school. If you are fortunate, your school may provide you with an interview itinerary prior to the interview, which will outline the amount of time allocated to each section of the interview. In one of my interviews, the itinerary listed all the professors who would be interviewing me. Armed with this information, I dedicated time to familiarize myself with their contributions, which greatly impressed them. In fact, one professor expressed gratitude as no one had ever taken the time to learn about them before. It is also worth finding out who the acting Dean is at your prospective school and whether the school actively engages on social media platforms. Remember, during the interview, you should also be evaluating the committee.

2. *Practice Makes Perfect!*

Practicing answering interview questions can truly make a difference. I still recall my experience during my first simulated interview when I was still in pre-med. I had always been accustomed to answering the common "Tell Me About Yourself" questions effortlessly, so when I was asked about personal aspects, I responded without much difficulty. However, as the interview progressed and focused on my pursuit of medicine, questions pertaining about the school I planned to apply to, ethical dilemmas, and my long-term impact in the field, I found myself taken aback. My confidence wavered, and I stumbled through each question, taking an excessive amount of time to answer. It felt as though I was under intense scrutiny. After that mock interview, I realized that I could never underestimate the importance of being prepared and requesting mock interviews for school. Around the same time, a dear friend of mine was also preparing for a medical school interview. He had applied to only one school, and I felt a deep responsibility to assist him. Nobody was more deserving than him! Two days before his interview, we met over Zoom (as it was during the COVID era) for an hour-long mock interview session. From discussing his childhood to exploring his motivation for pursuing medicine, and even handling questions about challenging classmates and ethical dilemmas, I appreciated his genuine responses. It was his compassion and selflessness that truly stood out. Most importantly, it was his unwavering determination. Through my friend, I not only shared the insights I gained from my own mock interview experience, but also learned valuable lessons by facilitating his mock interview.

My inquiry to you is how determined you are to pursue this opportunity? Are you committed to investing the effort required to practice diligently? Although there exists a wide range of interview questions, certain ones are more commonly asked than others. How well-versed are you in the field? Have you read the APhA's Pharmacy Today publication? Can you name any new medications you are familiar with and discuss the trending topics in pharmacy currently? Your interviewers will inquire about your background and experiences to gain a more detailed understanding of your skills and problem-solving abilities. Additionally, you might be prompted to talk about the most recent pharmacy article you have read. It is crucial not only to explain your motivation for choosing pharmacy but also to showcase relevant experiences and skills. Prior to my decision to pursue pharmacy, I had a background in mental health, where I gained extensive knowledge of psychiatric medications. I also conducted research and was published on Direct Oral Anticoagulant Therapy.

Many prospective pharmacy school applicants are attracted to the profession due to their desire to care for others, so demonstrate that passion! It is advantageous if you have engaged in work experience, networking, or conversations with industry professionals beforehand - this illustrates your understanding of the field and allows you to address both its challenges and rewards during the interview. While you do not necessarily need prior pharmacy work experience, sharing stories or anecdotes about relevant experiences can strengthen your responses.

Please refrain from discussing unrelated professions and instead, focus on highlighting the aspects of pharmacy that captivate you the most to showcase your academic interest. Remember to convey your enthusiasm throughout the interview process, whether it is a one-on-one interview, multiple mini-interviews (MMIs), or group discussions. During my pharmacy school interview, I encountered various types of questions such as stoichiometry questions and timed essay questions, which allowed me to demonstrate my professional writing skills and critical thinking abilities. Additionally, I participated in group discussions to address ethical dilemmas and engaged in panel interviews. While each interview may differ, practicing your responses to potential questions, whether it be in front of a mirror or with a family member, can greatly assist you in preparing for the interview.

3. Be Professional!

It is essential to emphasize the significance of professionalism. Please ensure that you dress appropriately for your interview. If possible, consider the colors you wear and avoid bright ones. Additionally, limit the amount of jewelry you wear. Depending on whether your interview is in person or virtual, wear comfortable dress shoes (if in person, you may even do a campus tour). Even if your interview is virtual, it is important to play the part and dress as if you were in person. I have heard stories of interview committees requiring interviewees to present themselves virtually. Therefore, it is crucial that you are punctual. Most likely, there will be a waiting room, so joining 10-15 minutes ahead of time allows you to address any issues before the interview. Test your connection beforehand, whether your interview will take place through teams, Google Meets, or Zoom. Please ensure that you download or update the necessary software in advance. Make sure your internet connection is strong and choose an area with limited distractions and noise for your interview.

During the interview, demonstrate good body language and maintain eye contact. Some interviews can be lengthy and require a significant amount of energy, so it is important to get a good night's sleep beforehand. Your interviewers will be able to gauge your engagement through your nonverbal cues, so be sure to actively listen and communicate effectively. Show enthusiasm and passion for the field of pharmacy. Although we have already discussed the importance of researching the school, take a final look at the school's mission statement before the interview. Prior to my own interviews, I would briefly review the school's website and take note of things that interested me for potential questions. I also made copies of my CV and publication, and even glanced over them before my interviews in case any questions were asked.

Rest assured that your unique qualities and experiences have caught the attention of your potential school, leading to your invitation for an interview. Trust in yourself and recognize that you are already highly regarded because of your background and personal story. The interview presents a chance for you to shine and make a lasting impression. It is an opportunity to convey your strengths and accomplishments through words, so be authentic, genuine, and maintain a professional demeanor. With these qualities, you are bound to excel in the interview and leave a lasting impact.

11.   Accepted

Receiving your first acceptance can be an overwhelming experience. If you're anything like me, you might find it hard to believe at first. I remember crying tears of joy when I received mine. I had applied to 12 schools in California and was quite anxious throughout the process. Spending almost 5 years at a community college before transferring to a 4-year institution, I had worked hard to get to this point. After completing my undergraduate degree, I pursued a master's in biomedical sciences, and reaching this milestone felt indescribable. However, once you're accepted, you start questioning if you've done enough to deserve it, **don't do that!**

The application process brought about a range of emotions, and I was hopeful to receive acceptance from at least one pharmacy school. After receiving multiple interview invitations and acceptances, I carefully chose the school that felt like home to me. It's important to remember that opinions may vary, so when you have multiple acceptances (which I hope for you), choose the school where you feel most comfortable and most supported. My decision was based on several factors, and I encourage you to consider what is important for your success in your doctoral program and make it nonnegotiable.

It is a significant achievement to gain admission to pharmacy school, and reaching this point likely involved a considerable amount of hard work and commitment. The foundation for the academic and practical experiences that pharmacy school will offer over the next three-to-four years has been laid by the courses completed during undergraduate studies. To ensure that your time in pharmacy school meets your expectations, it is crucial to prepare in advance as you get ready for this new phase in your life!

Relaxation. I understand that the journey to pharmacy school can be overwhelming, as I have experienced it myself. Before diving into the rigorous coursework and demanding schedule, it is important to take some time to unwind and recharge. This period of relaxation is crucial for your mental and emotional well-being.

During this time, it is important to prioritize spending quality moments with yourself and your loved ones. Engage in activities that bring you joy and help you discover new passions. Whether it is reading a book, going for a walk-in nature, or pursuing a hobby, make sure to allocate time for activities that bring you happiness and fulfillment.

Additionally, getting sufficient rest is essential before starting pharmacy school. Take this opportunity to establish a healthy sleep routine and ensure you are well-rested. Adequate rest will not only improve your overall well-being but also enhance your ability to focus and retain information during your classes.

I want you to know that I understand the overwhelming nature of this experience. The anticipation and excitement mixed with the nerves and uncertainties can be quite daunting. However, by taking the time to unwind and prioritize self-care, you are setting yourself up for success in pharmacy school. Remember to be kind to yourself and enjoy this period of relaxation before embarking on your educational journey.

Deposit. Additionally, it is important to consider the deadline for submitting your deposit. Many institutions have specific dates by which the deposit must be received to secure your spot. It is crucial to mark this date on your calendar and ensure that you submit the deposit on time to avoid any complications or potential loss of your acceptance.

Furthermore, it is worth researching if the deposit is refundable or non-refundable. Some institutions may have a non-refundable deposit policy, meaning that if you later decide not to attend the school, you will not be able to get your deposit back. This is an important factor to consider, especially if you are still unsure about your final decision.

In addition to the deposit, there may be other financial considerations to keep in mind. For example, some institutions may require you to submit a financial aid application or provide proof of funds to cover tuition and other expenses. It is important to familiarize yourself with these requirements and ensure that you meet them in a timely manner.

If you are concerned about the cost of the deposit, there are resources available to help. Many institutions offer financial aid or scholarships specifically for deposit fees. It is worth exploring these options and reaching out to the financial aid office for assistance. They may be able to provide guidance or offer alternative solutions to help alleviate the financial burden.

Lastly, it is important to remember that the deposit fee should not hinder your future progress. If you are truly passionate about attending a particular institution, do not let the deposit fee discourage you. There are often ways to work around financial constraints, such as payment plans or scholarships. It is important to communicate with the admissions committee and explore all available options to ensure that you can secure your spot without compromising your financial stability.

Professional Social Media Accounts. Having a professional social media account, especially in the pharmacy field, can provide numerous benefits and opportunities. One platform that is highly recommended for professionals is LinkedIn. Creating a LinkedIn profile allows you to showcase your education, skills, and experience, making it easier for potential employers or colleagues to find and connect with you.

LinkedIn also offers various groups and communities specifically tailored to the pharmacy industry. Joining these groups can provide you with a platform to engage in discussions, share knowledge, and learn from experienced professionals. By actively participating in these groups, you can establish yourself as a knowledgeable and engaged individual in the field.

Instagram and Twitter, although more commonly associated with personal use, can also be valuable tools for pharmacy professionals. These platforms allow you to share insights, articles, and resources related to the pharmacy field. By consistently posting relevant content, you can position yourself as a thought leader and attract a following of like-minded individuals.

Networking is a crucial aspect of any profession, and social media platforms provide an excellent opportunity to expand your professional circle. By connecting with fellow pharmacy students and professionals, you can build relationships that may lead to job opportunities, mentorship, or collaborations. Additionally, networking can expose you to different perspectives and ideas, helping you stay informed about industry trends and advancements.

Furthermore, having a professional social media account allows you to inspire and guide others who may be seeking advice or guidance in the pharmacy field. By sharing your experiences, successes, and challenges, you can motivate and support aspiring pharmacists. This not only helps others but also enhances your own professional reputation and credibility.

Mental Preparation. During this time, it is also important to mentally prepare yourself for the challenges that lie ahead. Pharmacy school can be demanding and rigorous, so it is essential to cultivate a positive mindset and develop effective study habits. Setting realistic goals and creating a study schedule can help you stay organized and focused throughout your academic journey.

Additionally, it is beneficial to familiarize yourself with the pharmacy profession and stay informed about current trends and developments in the field (can't stress this enough). This will not only enhance your understanding of the curriculum but also prepare you for future career opportunities.

As you embark on this new chapter, remember to stay motivated and persevere through any obstacles that may come your way. With dedication, hard work, and a positive attitude, you can successfully navigate through pharmacy school and achieve your goals.

Background Checks. It is important to be proactive and organized when it comes to fulfilling these requirements, as they are essential for your enrollment in the program. Make sure to plan and give yourself enough time to gather all the necessary documents and complete any required steps. This will help you avoid any last-minute stress or complications that could potentially delay your enrollment.

If you have any questions or concerns about the background check, drug screening, or immunization requirements, don't hesitate to reach out to your school's admissions office or healthcare provider for guidance. They will be able to provide you with the necessary information and support to ensure that you are fully prepared for enrollment.

Remember that these requirements are in place to ensure the safety and well-being of all students and staff within the school community. By taking the time to fulfill these obligations in a timely manner, you are not only demonstrating your commitment to your education but also showing respect for the policies and procedures put in place by the school.

12. Notes

Prescription for Success

Notes

Prescription for Success

Notes

Prescription for Success

Notes

Prescription for Success

Notes

Prescription for Success

IV. Ask and It Shall be Given, Seek and You Shall Find

13. Scholarships and Financial Aid

Numerous scholarships and financial aid options exist to support students in pharmacy school. The most prevalent forms of financial assistance are typically awarded according to academic achievements and personal financial situations.

Scholarships Based on Merit. Scholarships based on merit are awarded to students who have demonstrated exceptional academic achievements, effective leadership skills, active participation in volunteer activities, and engagement in various extracurricular pursuits. These scholarships are highly competitive and are typically granted to individuals who have excelled in multiple areas of their academic and personal lives.

To be eligible for such scholarships, students must have a strong academic record, often maintaining a specific grade point average (GPA). This requirement ensures that recipients continue to prioritize their studies and maintain their academic excellence even after receiving the scholarship.

In addition to academic achievements, scholarship committees also consider a student's leadership abilities. This includes holding leadership positions in student organizations, clubs, or community groups, as well as demonstrating effective communication, problem-solving, and decision-making skills. By recognizing and rewarding students with strong leadership potential, these scholarships aim to encourage and support the development of future leaders in various fields.

Furthermore, active involvement in volunteer activities is another important criterion for merit-based scholarships. Students who have dedicated their time and efforts to serving their communities, whether through local charities, non-profit organizations, or community service projects, are highly regarded by scholarship committees. This involvement showcases a student's commitment to making a positive impact on society and demonstrates their willingness to contribute to the betterment of their community.

Engagement in extracurricular pursuits is also taken into consideration when awarding merit-based scholarships. Students who have participated in sports, arts, music, debate, or other activities outside of their academic curriculum are seen as well-rounded individuals who have developed a range of skills and interests. These pursuits showcase a student's ability to manage their time effectively, work collaboratively with others, and pursue their passions beyond the classroom.

It is important to note that maintaining eligibility for these scholarships often requires recipients to uphold a specific GPA throughout their academic journey. This requirement ensures that students continue to prioritize their studies and strive for academic excellence even after receiving the scholarship. By setting this expectation, scholarship committees aim to support students in their educational pursuits and encourage them to continue their commitment to academic success.

Scholarships Based on Financial Need. The need-based scholarships are designed to provide financial support to students who are facing financial difficulties in paying for their education. These scholarships aim to ensure that students from low-income backgrounds have equal access to educational opportunities and can pursue their academic goals without being burdened by financial constraints.

To determine the amount of financial assistance that a student requires, they must complete and submit a Free Application for Federal Student Aid (FAFSA). The FAFSA is a comprehensive form that collects information about the student's and their family's financial situation, including income, assets, and expenses. This information is then used to calculate the Expected Family Contribution (EFC), which is the amount that the student and their family are expected to contribute towards their education.

Based on the EFC, the financial aid office at the educational institution evaluates the student's eligibility for need-based scholarships. The office takes into consideration various factors such as tuition fees, living expenses, and other educational costs to determine the amount of financial assistance required by the student.

The need-based scholarships can cover a range of expenses, including tuition fees, textbooks, housing, and other educational expenses. The amount of financial assistance provided may vary depending on the student's financial need, the availability of funds, and the specific criteria set by the scholarship program.

By offering need-based scholarships, educational institutions aim to make education more accessible and affordable for students who may not have the financial means to pursue higher education. These scholarships not only alleviate the financial burden on students but also enable them to focus on their studies and achieve their academic goals without worrying about the cost of education.

Scholarships Promoting Diversity. Diversity scholarships aim to promote inclusivity and equal opportunities for minority and underrepresented students. These scholarships recognize the importance of diversity and seek to address the underrepresentation of certain groups.

One of the key factors considered when granting diversity scholarships is the student's racial and/or ethnic background. This is because historically marginalized racial and ethnic groups have faced barriers to accessing higher education, including pharmacy programs. By providing scholarships specifically for these students, pharmacy schools, for instance, aim to increase representation and diversity within the profession.

Gender is another factor that may be considered when awarding diversity scholarships. For example, though the pharmacy profession has seen an increase in the number of women in recent years, there is still a gender disparity in certain areas of pharmacy practice. Scholarships targeting female students help to address this imbalance and encourage more women to pursue careers in pharmacy.

Age can also be a consideration for diversity scholarships. Some scholarships may be specifically designed for non-traditional students, such as those who are returning to school after a gap in their education or those who are pursuing a second career. These scholarships recognize the unique challenges faced by older students and provide financial support to help them achieve their educational goals.

In some cases, religious affiliations may also be considered when awarding diversity scholarships. This is particularly relevant in cases where certain religious communities are underrepresented in a profession. Scholarships that consider religious affiliations aim to create a more inclusive environment for students from diverse religious backgrounds.

Pharmacy schools are typically the primary source of these diversity scholarships. Students are encouraged to directly contact the schools they are interested in attending to explore scholarship options. The schools can provide information on the specific scholarships available, eligibility criteria, and application processes. Additionally, students may also find resources and information on external organizations or foundations that offer diversity scholarships in pharmacy education.

More Scholarship Opportunities. Scholarship opportunities are widely available, particularly for those pursuing further education through continuing education, graduate residency programs, and professional development. Additionally, numerous national, state, and local pharmacy organizations offer scholarships, making it crucial for students to research the criteria and number of scholarships provided by these organizations.

Apart from scholarships, government grants and loans serve as alternative sources of financial aid. While grants do not require repayment, loans must be repaid with interest. The amount of financial aid and the type of loans offered to students are typically determined based on the cost of attendance and the financial background of the student and their family. It is worth noting that federal loans generally offer more favorable terms and conditions compared to private loans, such as deferred payments until after graduation and various repayment plans.

Given the wide range of scholarships and financial aid available, students have numerous options to explore. It is highly recommended for students to begin researching and applying for scholarships as early as possible. Applying for all eligible scholarships and meeting deadlines is crucial to maximize opportunities and alleviate financial burdens. Seeking guidance from academic advisors and financial aid advisors can provide valuable information and advice on different scholarships. Lastly, students should strive to create a strong application, including well-crafted essays and an updated resume highlighting leadership and volunteer experiences.

14. Housing

Once you have enrolled in a school, it is highly recommended to initiate your search for housing without delay. It is always wiser to exercise caution rather than face regret later. The least desirable situation would be to begin your housing search merely 1-2 months before your program commences, as you will already have a multitude of tasks to accomplish. To alleviate the stress of transitioning, certain schools may provide resources to assist students in finding suitable housing. Drawing from my personal experience, schools may utilize social media platforms such as Facebook and Instagram to facilitate connections between new and current students. In certain instances, you may even come across members of the admissions team who offer rooms or homes for rent to students, as they comprehend the challenges associated with securing housing for newcomers.

It can also be beneficial to reach out to current students or alumni of the school to get their insights and recommendations on housing options. They can provide valuable information about the neighborhoods, safety, transportation, and other factors to consider when choosing a place to live.

Furthermore, it is essential to set a budget for housing expenses and stick to it. Consider not only the monthly rent but also additional costs such as utilities, internet, and transportation. It is crucial to have a clear understanding of the financial commitment involved in renting a place.

When visiting potential housing options, make sure to ask questions about the lease terms, maintenance responsibilities, and any additional fees or restrictions. It is important to have a clear understanding of the rental agreement before signing any contracts.

In some cases, it may be beneficial to consider roommate options to share the cost of living and create a sense of community. However, it is crucial to establish clear expectations and boundaries with roommates to ensure a harmonious living environment.

Lastly, it is advisable to start the housing search early to have enough time to visit different options, negotiate terms, and make an informed decision. Rushing into a housing agreement without proper research can lead to regrets and unnecessary stress.

Remember, finding suitable housing when enrolling in a school requires proactive planning and research. By utilizing resources provided by the school, exploring various platforms, seeking recommendations, and considering important factors such as location and budget, students can secure a comfortable and suitable living arrangement for their academic journey.

15.   Pharmacy Career Options

Prior to embarking on my journey in pharmacy, my knowledge was limited to retail pharmacy. I was unaware of the vast array of different career paths available to pharmacists. While some may envision themselves working in a local pharmacy, dispensing medication, and offering healthcare advice, it is crucial to recognize the diverse range of opportunities that exist for pharmacists. These alternative paths may necessitate further education, or training beyond obtaining a PharmD.

Some of the alternative career paths for pharmacists include working in pharmaceutical research and development, regulatory affairs, clinical trials, drug safety monitoring, medication therapy management, managed care, public health, academia, consulting, and even entrepreneurship. Each of these career paths offers unique challenges and opportunities for pharmacists to make a difference in the healthcare industry.

For example, pharmacists working in pharmaceutical research and development play a crucial role in developing new medications and improving existing ones. They may work in collaboration with scientists, physicians, and other healthcare professionals to conduct clinical trials, analyze data, and ensure the safety and efficacy of medications.

Pharmacists in regulatory affairs are responsible for ensuring that pharmaceutical products meet regulatory requirements set by government agencies such as the Food and Drug Administration (FDA). They may work on submitting applications for new drug approvals, monitoring compliance with regulations, and communicating with regulatory authorities.

Clinical pharmacists work directly with patients and healthcare providers to optimize medication therapy and improve patient outcomes. They may work in hospitals, clinics, or other healthcare settings to provide medication management services, conduct medication reviews, and educate patients about their medications.

Pharmacists in managed care organizations play a key role in managing medication costs, improving medication adherence, and ensuring quality care for patients. They may work on formulary management, medication utilization reviews, and medication therapy management programs to help patients get the most benefit from their medications.

In academia, pharmacists may work as professors, researchers, or administrators in colleges of pharmacy or other educational institutions. They may teach pharmacy students, conduct research in various areas of pharmacy practice, and contribute to the advancement of the profession through scholarly activities.

In general, the pharmacy sector provides pharmacists with a diverse array of career paths to consider and follow. A variety of roles and specializations can be found in the upcoming pages. Pharmacists can significantly contribute to patient care, drug advancement, healthcare regulations, and public health by broadening their expertise and abilities beyond conventional retail pharmacy practices.

Roles in Academic Pharmacy - *Careers in academia within the field of pharmacy usually involve educating and preparing aspiring pharmacists. These positions demand a strong foundation in pharmacy as well as a genuine enthusiasm for teaching.*

The following is a list of potential options:

Clinical Rotations Preceptor

Education & Training Pharmacist

Lecturer

Licensing Exam Preceptor

Pharmaceutics Professor

Pharmacodynamics Researcher

Pharmacokinetics Researcher

Pharmacology Researcher

Pharmacy Practice Researcher

Pharmacy Student Mentor

Research & Development Pharmacist

Residency

Teacher Practitioner

Teaching Assistant

Teaching Fellow

Therapeutics Professor

Roles in Specialty Pharmacy Practice - *The career paths within this category are some of the most prevalent career choices for pharmacists. Typically, they provide chances for hands-on patient care in various clinical environments.*

The following is a list of potential options:

Ambulatory Care Pharmacist

Aseptic Infusion

Bariatrics Pharmacist

Biologics Pharmacist

Chief Pharmaceutical Officer

Clinical Director

Clinical Pharmacist

Clinical Programs Leader

Community Pharmacist

Compounding Pharmacist

Cosmetics Pharmacist

Critical Care Pharmacist

Director of Clinical Solutions

Emergency Care Pharmacist

Functional Medicine Pharmacist

General Practice Pharmacist

Geriatrics Pharmacist

Home Care Pharmacist

Home Health Equipment

Hormone Medicine Pharmacist

Hospital Pharmacist

Immunization Pharmacist

Infectious Disease Pharmacy

Infectious Disease Testing Pharmacist Management Roles

Internal Medicine

Long-Term Care Operations Pharmacist

Managed Care Pharmacist

Mental Health & Addictions Pharmacist

Herbal Medicine Pharmacist

Nutraceutical Pharmacist

Oncology Pharmacist

Outpatient Pharmacist

Pain Management

Pediatric Pharmacist

Pharmacy Manager

Regulatory Health Project Leader

Sexual Health Pharmacist

Surgical Care Pharmacist

Systemic Therapy Pharmacist

Travel Medicine Pharmacist

Veterinary Pharmacist

Roles in the Pharmaceutical Industry - *Pharmacy professions falling under this category are ideal for individuals possessing extensive knowledge in medications and a profound inclination towards business or research.*

The following is a list of potential options:

Biomedical Researcher

Clinical Research Associate

Digital Diagnostics Researcher

Digital Therapeutics Researcher

Drug Safety Associate

Forensic Scientist

Industrial Manufacturing

Marketing & Medical Strategy

Medical Science Liaison

Medicinal Chemist

Pharmaceutical Modeler

Pharmaceutical Sales Representative

Pharmaceutical Scientist

Pharmaceutical Study

Pharmacist Clinical Pathologist

Pharmacologist

Pharmacovigilance Specialist

Product Development

Quality Assurance

Quality Control Chemist

Regulatory Affairs Pharmacist

Regulatory Affairs Specialist

Research Scientist

Toxicology Pharmacist

Roles in Pharmacy Within the Field of Technology and Health Informatics - *Individuals interested in healthcare records, data, or systems might find pharmacy positions within the technology and health informatics field appealing.*

The following is a list of potential options:

Automation Pharmacist

Clinical Applications Pharmacist

Clinical Data Analyst

Clinical Software Development Specialist

Clinical Software Integration Specialist

Clinical Solutions Pharmacist

Digital Health Specialist

Electronic Health Record Training Pharmacist

Health Informatics Specialist

Information Technology Pharmacist

Pharmacy Informatics Specialist

Social Media Engagement

Telehealth Service Provider

Virtual Clinical Pharmacist

Roles of Government and Regulation - *Government officials and regulatory pharmacists can utilize their extensive knowledge in medications to provide valuable insights for government regulations, establish effective policies and protocols, guarantee the well-being of patients, and fulfill various other responsibilities.*

The following is a list of potential options:

Clinical Inspection Pharmacist

Consumer Safety Officer

Correctional Facility Pharmacist

Drug Advertising Reviewer

Drug Pricing Reviewer

Drug Reimbursement Expert

Drug Safety Data Reviewer

Medicines Advisor

Military Pharmacist

Nuclear Pharmacist

Patient Advocacy Board Member

Pharmaceutical Services Commissioner

Pharmacoeconomics Specialist

Pharmacy Advocacy Member

Pharmacy Education Accreditation Reviewer

Poison Control Pharmacist

Public Health Service Pharmacist

Regulatory Board Member

Specialist Pharmaceutical Advisor to Local, Regional, or National Government

Alternative Pharmacy Career Paths - *Pharmacists are involved in a wide range of industries, showcasing their versatility and expertise.*

The following is a list of potential options:

Academic Detailer

Aerospace

Business Adviser

Career Development Coach

Central Fill Pharmacist

Continuing Education Provider

Digital Therapeutics Specialist

Drug Information Pharmacist

Estate & Tax Planning Consultant

Geospatial Pharmacist

Life Coach

Medical Writer

Medication Safety Management Specialist

Pharmacogenomics Specialist

Pharmacy Financial Consultant

Pharmacy Programs Coordinator

Pharmacy Research Coordinator

Pharmacy Strategy Consultant

Start-Up Developer

Supply Chain Pharmacist

Visit PharmacyForMe.org to learn more about these endless opportunities.

16. Notes

Prescription for Success

Notes

Prescription for Success

Notes

Prescription for Success

Notes

Prescription for Success

Notes

Prescription for Success

V. Discover the Possibilities to Become the Person You Aspire to Be

17.   Recommended Pharmacy Resources

Whether you are currently in the process of applying or preparing to start your program, there are several pharmacy resources that come highly recommended to support you along the way. It is suggested to start by finding a mentor in the pharmacy field, regardless of your academic or professional background. Connecting with a mentor can offer valuable insights and guidance to help you get ready for interviews and excel in your program. Based on my personal experience, I found it beneficial to stay informed about industry advancements through reading pharmacy articles. Moreover, I utilized social media platforms such as Instagram and LinkedIn, and subscribed to Pharmacy Times, to enhance my understanding of various topics, including controversial medications and the challenges encountered by underserved communities.

Moreover, I revisited stoichiometry and practiced conversion problems based on a friend's recommendation, anticipating chemistry-related questions during interviews. Joining pre-pharmacy clubs can also be advantageous in familiarizing yourself with commonly prescribed drugs, allowing you to understand the key characteristics of medications used in various healthcare settings. Exploring websites that offer detailed information on brand names, pharmacologic categories, dosage forms, administration methods, contraindications, drug interactions, and adverse effects can further enhance your knowledge. Remember, as a pharmacist, you hold expertise in medications, so taking advantage of these resources early on can give you a competitive advantage.

18. Prescription Drugs Worth Memorizing

Generic Name	Trade Name	General Category	Therapeutic (Drug) Classification
Amoxicillin/ Clavulanate potassium	Augmentin	Anti-infective	Penicillin antibiotic
Metronidazole	Vandazole, Metrogel, Flagyl	Anti-infective	Antiprotozoal, Antibacterial
Amoxicillin	Trimox, Moxatag, Amoxil	Anti-infective	Penicillin antibiotic
Cephalexin	Keflex	Anti-infective	Cephalosporin
Azithromycin	Zithromax Z-Pak, AzaSite, Zmax	Anti-infective	Macrolide antibiotic
Fluconazole	Diflucan	Anti-infective	Antifungal
Doxycycline hyclate	Targadox, Vibramycin, Acticlate, Doryx	Anti-infective	Tetracycline antibiotic
Lisinopril/ Lis/Hydrochlorothiazide (HCTZ)	Prinivil, Zestril	Cardiovascular	Antihypertensive, ACE inhibitor, Zestoretic combo w/ diuretic
Amlodipine	Norvasc	Cardiovascular	Calcium channel blocker
Atorvastatin	Lipitor	Cardiovascular	HMG-CoA reductase inhibitor, Antihyperlipidemic
Losartan/Los/HCTZ	Cozaar, Hyzaar	Cardiovascular	ARB Antihypertensive
Metoprolol succinate ER	Toprol XL	Cardiovascular	Beta blocker (Beta-1 selective)
Hydrochlorothiazide	Microzide, Oretic	Cardiovascular	Thiazide diuretic
Simvastatin	Zocor	Cardiovascular	HMG-CoA reductase inhibitor, Antihyperlipidemic
Rosuvastatin	Crestor	Cardiovascular	HMG-CoA reductase inhibitor, Antihyperlipidemic
Furosemide	Lasix	Cardiovascular	Loop diuretic

Spironolactone	Aldactone	Cardiovascular	Potassium-sparing diuretic
Lisinopril/Hydrochlorothiazide	Zestoretic	Cardiovascular	ACE inhibitor, Antihypertensive
Metoprolol tartrate	Lopressor	Cardiovascular	Beta blocker (Beta-1 selective)
Acetaminophen hydrocodone	Vicodin, Lortab, Lorcet	CNS	Analgesic, Antipyretic opioid
Amphetamine/Dextroamphetamine	Adderall, Adderall XR	CNS	Stimulant, treat ADD
Gabapentin	Horizant, Neurontin	CNS	Antiepileptic, Neuropathic analgesic
Trazodone	Desyrel, Oleptro	CNS	Antidepressant
Escitalopram oxalate	Lexapro	CNS	SSRI - Antidepressant
Fluoxetine	Prozac, Sarafem	CNS	SSRI - Antidepressant
Zolpidem tartrate	Ambien	CNS	Sedative hypnotic
Bupropion ER	Wellbutrin, Zyban, Forfivo, Aplenzin	CNS	Antidepressant, Smoking cessation aid
Methocarbamol	Robaxin	CNS	Muscle relaxant
Clonazepam	Klonopin	CNS	Benzodiazepine
Sertraline	Zoloft	CNS	SSRI-Antidepressant
Ondansetron	Zofran	CNS	5-HT3 Receptor antagonist
Phenobarbital	Luminal, Solfoton	CNS	Antiepileptic, hypnotic
Meloxicam	Mobic	CNS	NSAID
Cyclobenzaprine	Flexeril, Fexmid, Amirex	CNS	Muscle relaxant
Ibuprofen	Advil, Motrin	CNS	NSAID
Alprazolam	Xanax	CNS	Benzodiazepine
Estradiol	Estrace, Climara, Minivelle	Endocrine	Estrogen hormone
Methylprednisolone	Medrol	Endocrine	Steroid, anti-inflammatory
Metformin	Glucophage, Riomet	Endocrine	Antidiabetic (Biguanide)

Levothyroxine	Synthroid, Levo-T, Tirosint, Unithroid, Levoxyl	Endocrine	Thyroid hormone (T4)
Prednisone	Rayos, Deltasone, Prednicort, Orasone	Endocrine	Corticosteroid (anti-inflammatory)
Omeprazole	Prilosec	Gastrointestinal	Proton pump inhibitor
Pantoprazole sodium	Protonix	Gastrointestinal	Proton pump inhibitor
Famotidine	Pepcid, Pepcid AC, Zantac 360	Gastrointestinal	H2-Antihistamine
Sildenafil citrate	Viagra, Revatio	Genitourinary	Erectile dysfunction - Vasodilator
Tadalafil	Cialis	Genitourinary	Erectile dysfunction - Vasodilator
Albuterol	Ventolin HFA, Proair HFA, Proventil HFA	Respiratory	Anti-asthmatic - Leukotriene inhibitor
Benzonatate	Tessalon Perles, Zonatuss	Respiratory	Local anesthetic, non-narcotic alternative
Cetirizine	Zyrtec	Respiratory	Antihistamine
Fluticasone	Flonase	Respiratory	Allergic rhinitis - Nasal steroid

19. Oath of a Pharmacist

The AACP Board of Directors and APhA Board of Trustees, as the governing bodies of the American Association of Colleges of Pharmacy and the American Pharmacists Association respectively, play a crucial role in shaping the profession of pharmacy. One of their responsibilities is to periodically review and revise the Oath of a Pharmacist, a document that outlines the ethical principles and responsibilities that pharmacists should uphold.

The Oath of a Pharmacist is widely adopted by pharmacy schools and institutions across the United States. It serves as a guiding framework for pharmacists, reminding them of their commitment to provide safe and effective patient care. By incorporating the Oath into their academic years, pharmacy schools ensure that their students are aware of the ethical standards expected of them upon graduation.

Furthermore, it is essential for graduates to take the Oath of a Pharmacist as they enter the profession. By reciting the Oath, they publicly declare their dedication to upholding the values and principles of the pharmacy profession. This act not only reinforces their commitment to ethical conduct but also serves as a reminder of the responsibilities they have towards their patients and the community.

The Oath of a Pharmacist encompasses various commitments that pharmacists must adhere to throughout their professional journey. It emphasizes the importance of maintaining professional conduct, which includes practicing with integrity, honesty, and respect for patients and colleagues. Pharmacists are also encouraged to advocate for patient care, ensuring that their patients receive the best possible treatment and outcomes.

Additionally, the Oath recognizes the role of pharmacists in nurturing the future generation of pharmacists. It highlights the importance of mentoring and supporting aspiring pharmacists, fostering a culture of continuous learning and professional development. By doing so, pharmacists contribute to the growth and advancement of the pharmacy profession.

Moreover, the Oath of a Pharmacist places a strong emphasis on the values of equity, inclusion, and diversity. It urges pharmacists to actively promote health equity, ensuring that all patients have equal access to healthcare services and resources. Pharmacists are encouraged to advocate for underserved populations and work towards eliminating healthcare disparities. By embracing diversity and inclusion, pharmacists can create a more inclusive and equitable healthcare system.

"I promise to devote myself to a lifetime of service to others through the profession of pharmacy. In fulfilling this vow:

- I will consider the welfare of humanity and relief of suffering my primary concerns.

- I will promote inclusion, embrace diversity, and advocate for justice to advance health equity.

- I will apply my knowledge, experience, and skills to the best of my ability to assure optimal outcomes for all patients.

- I will respect and protect all personal and health information entrusted to me.

- I will accept the responsibility to improve my professional knowledge, expertise, and self-awareness.

- I will hold myself and my colleagues to the highest principles of our profession's moral, ethical, and legal conduct.

- I will embrace and advocate changes that improve patient care.

- I will utilize my knowledge, skills, experiences, and values to prepare the next generation of pharmacists.

I take these vows voluntarily with the full realization of the responsibility with which I am entrusted by the public."

Be sure to visit pharmacist.com (APhA) for more information.

20. Notes

Prescription for Success

Notes

Prescription for Success

Notes

Prescription for Success

Notes

Prescription for Success

Notes

Prescription for Success

Acknowledgements

I am deeply grateful to my Lord and Savior Jesus Christ, who walks beside me, demonstrates His love, provides support, and shows me that He is in control of my life. By staying close to Him, I trust that He will fulfill the desires of my heart. I also want to express my appreciation to the individuals who have crossed my path through God's guidance, offering help, encouragement, support, and friendship.

Reflecting on my journey and the sacrifices made, I am moved by the kindness of friends, family, and even strangers who wish me well. I acknowledge each person I have encountered and look forward to meeting those who I hope to inspire in the future, just as I have been inspired by others.

Jeremiah 29:11

About the Author

First and foremost, I would like to express my gratitude for your support. Prior to sharing a little more about me I sincerely pray for an abundance of success in your life. Furthermore, I hope and pray that you have discovered at least one valuable aspect within this book that can be applicable to your own journey.

Growing up underrepresented and being the first in my family to pursue higher education, I must admit that this journey has been exceptionally challenging for me. I often found myself feeling lost and overlooked. This is precisely why I felt compelled to write this book. My intention was to share my personal experiences throughout this process. I was born and raised in California and attended Charles R. Drew University of Medicine and Science, where I earned my bachelor's degree in biomedical science. Subsequently, I pursued my master's degree in biomedical sciences from California Baptist University, an institution that truly transformed my life.

Recently, I have not only discovered a passion for writing but have also self-published a few children's books. My aspiration is for my story to serve as an inspiration for others, demonstrating that they too can strive to achieve their dreams, regardless of their upbringing or circumstances.

In my leisure time, I enjoy visiting beaches, cherishing moments with my family, and indulging in the luxury of sleeping in whenever possible. My goal is to pursue a career in Psychiatric Pharmacy.

Thank you for being a part of this incredible journey with me.

Things I Wish I Knew

It is natural to have moments of self-doubt and to question our abilities, especially in a field as demanding and critical as healthcare. However, it is crucial to remind ourselves that we are more than our mistakes. Our worth is not defined by the errors we make, but rather by our resilience, determination, and willingness to learn and grow from those mistakes.

Learning not to be too harsh on ourselves is a valuable lesson that can positively impact our personal and professional lives. By acknowledging that we are human and bound to make mistakes, we can cultivate self-compassion and treat ourselves with kindness and understanding. This mindset allows us to approach challenges with a growth mindset, viewing setbacks as opportunities for growth and improvement rather than as reflections of our worth.

Understanding that we are more than our mistakes requires a shift in perspective. It involves recognizing that our worth is not solely determined by our achievements or the absence of mistakes, but rather by our inherent value as individuals. We are complex beings with unique talents, strengths, and qualities that extend far beyond any single error or setback.

In the healthcare field, it is easy to fall into the trap of imposter syndrome, feeling like we don't deserve to be in the positions we hold. However, it is important to remember that our journey and experiences have shaped us into the capable professionals we are today. Our dedication, hard work, and continuous learning have brought us to where we are, and we should take pride in that.

Having faith, can provide us with the reassurance and confidence we need to overcome self-doubt. Believing in something greater than ourselves can help us recognize that we are part of a larger plan and that our presence in our chosen field is not a coincidence. It can give us the strength to trust in our abilities and embrace the challenges that come our way.

Ultimately, I wish I knew the significance of treating myself with gentleness and acknowledging that I am more than my mistakes (a lifelong journey). This journey requires self-reflection, self-compassion, and a commitment to personal growth. By embracing my worth and recognizing my abilities, I can confidently navigate the healthcare field, knowing that I can overcome any obstacle and make a positive impact on the lives of others.

www.ingramcontent.com/pod-product-compliance
Lightning Source LLC
Chambersburg PA
CBHW070437130626
46553CB00006B/2222